Is Gluten Hiding in Your Kid's Things?

An **eZ** Guide for Raising Gluten-Free Kids; Including Lists of Gluten-Free Products for Children and Infants.

Marian Z Geringer
e*Z*GLUTEN-FREE LIFE

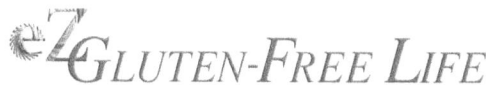
eZ GLUTEN-FREE LIFE

Additional Gluten-Free Handbooks Available:
By Marian Z Geringer

Gluten-Free Living 101
An eZ step by step guide on how to start living a successful gluten-free life today.

Is Gluten Hiding in Your Shampoo? It Was Hiding in Mine!
This handbook lets you know if gluten is hiding in over 2,500 personal care products. The list is divided by brand and type of product for easy reading.

Marian is currently working on **Is Gluten Hiding in Unexpected Places?**
Gluten can be found in products you may not have considered such as:

Alcoholic Drinks	Fast Foods
Candy	Sauces
Cleaning Products	Spices
Cooking Sprays	and More...

**Is Gluten Hiding in Your
Kid's Things?
A Kid's Products Handbook**

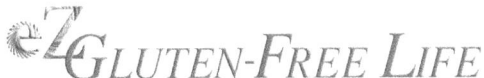

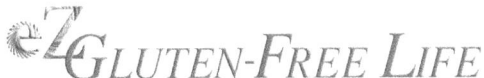GLUTEN-FREE LIFE

The handbook is divided into 2 sections.

Section 1: Pages 5 through 13 consist of brief definitions of gluten, a list where it can be found and a detailed list of ingredients found in cosmetics and body care products that contain gluten.

Section 2: Is an itemized list of personal care products and brands. Simply use the Table of Contents to direct you to the type of personal care product you are interested in and go to that page.

Example: page 40 is Kid's Sunscreen.

• All the brands are in alphabetical order.

• Under each brand's name is the products they carry.

• The list will tell you if the product is gluten-free (GF) or not.

• The far right column, labeled, "Company Information" provides you with the response I received directly from the company.

• Page 5 provides a list of key terms used.

Take this handbook with you to the store so that you can be confident that the products you are purchasing are safe. If you have any doubts, please contact the company directly. Companies are always revamping the lines, so please refer to their websites.

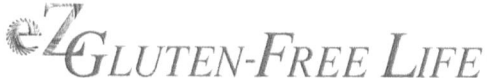
eZ Gluten-Free Life

Table of Contents

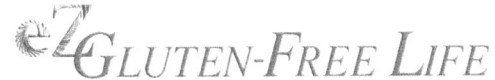
eZ Gluten-Free Life

Key Terms	Definitions
CC	Cross Contamination: Product may have been exposed to gluten during the manufacturing process.
Contact Company	Line is too extensive for the company to comment on ingredients in the products. It is necessary to contact the company about a specific product in the line.
Contains Oats	These products contain oats that are not gluten-free.
EXCEPT	The far right column will have the specific products that contain gluten.
GF	Gluten Free
GLUTEN	Definitely contains gluten
GLUTEN/CC	Product contains gluten or has been exposed to cross contamination.
Read Info	Read the company information in the far right column.
Read Labels	You will need to review the ingredients for this brands individual products.
Undetermined	Company does not have gluten information about the product.

Disclaimer:

Please remember this handbook is meant to be used as an informative guide and is in no way meant to replace or conflict with medical advice of physicians. Always check the labels, ingredients and allergen warnings before consuming any food product or using any product that may come in contact with your body. Ingredients and formulas can change at any time. Regulations vary from country to country, so products listed as gluten-free in the U.S. may not be gluten-free in other countries.

Many ingredient labels appear NOT to have gluten in them yet during the company's communication to me, the company either does not list them as gluten-free or they stated that the product has not been tested and/or certified gluten-free. This especially occurs with non- food products. I have listed these products as: "Contains no gluten ingredients but has not been tested for CC." (CC = Cross Contamination)

This handbook includes a large cross section of companies and brands. New companies and products are introduced continually and other products discontinued on a regular basis. This handbook is not an exhaustive list.

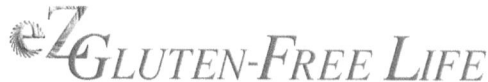

GLUTEN-FREE LIFE

Gluten is the topic of conversation these days. No matter where we turn gluten is being discussed. Until recently, there has been very little known about gluten related diseases. Accurate testing for Celiac has only been around since the early 1970's and gluten intolerance is only now being researched and understood.

All too often, once a patient is diagnosed, he/she is left to figure out what to do. I have observed that it takes many people, including myself, quite a while to put the pieces together. It is not from a lack of information; it is quite the opposite. The information pool is enormous and growing every day. There are books, websites, blogs, and seminars; just to mention a few resources. The internet is streaming with information about Celiac's disease. There is blog after blog discussing gluten, diseases related to gluten, and how to cook and bake gluten-free. The issue is that once a diagnosis is made a gluten-free lifestyle is required. The patient needs to implement the changes quickly in order to start the healing process. With so much information scattered in so many directions it can take months, even years, for the patient to find his/her way through it all.

Removing gluten from our children's world has its own set of concerns. Gluten and/or oats can be found in art supplies, diapers, children's shampoos, and other body care products, medications as well as infant and toddler foods.

This handbook will equip parents with clear and simple gluten-free product information. In addition, there are suggestions on how to find positive ways to approach the dietary changes. Educating our children about their specific diet needs will help them, so one day they can take care of their own dietary needs.

This handbook is dedicated to keeping our gluten-free children as safe as possible. The handbook has detailed product information and creative ideas to help the child adjust to this lifestyle change.

I have spent several years researching whether or not gluten can be found in certain brands and companies. I have compiled all the research into 3 additional handbooks. The handbooks are conveniently set up, so they can easily tuck in to a handbag or briefcase and/or carried into a store.

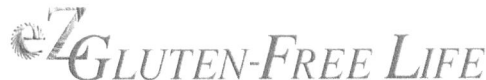
eZGLUTEN-FREE LIFE

TWELVE STEPS TO TRANSITIONING TO A GLUTEN-FREE LIFESTYLE:

1. Educate yourself: Use this handbook as the first step in the learning process. It has important information that will help you during the initial process.
2. Remember it is best to take this one step at a time and not get too overwhelmed.
3. Start by eliminating and replacing the basic gluten products.
4. Learn how to read labels so you can recognize gluten ingredients.
5. Go through the pantry, refrigerator and freezer to eliminate all gluten items.
6. Become familiar with gluten-free flours and brand names.
7. Create a grocery list of items that needs immediate replacing and go shopping.
8. Discover restaurants that offer gluten-free menus. Use apps and online sites.
9. Purchase gluten-free magazines to keep you up-to-date on the latest research, recipes and products.
10. As you become more comfortable start looking into concealed sources of gluten. Cross Contamination is important to avoid. Gluten is in many personal care products such as deodorant, dental products, hair products, etc.
11. Keep a POSITIVE ATTITUDE. Going gluten-free is the healthiest thing I have ever done. I now see it as a gift. I no longer suffer from a myriad of disorders and I do not need surgery or medication to feel this good. Everyone heals at different rates and times, so please be patient and take it one day at a time.
12. Connect with other people who are living gluten-free so you have someone to bounce ideas off of. Join a support group, read blogs, and just put it out there at work or school. You will be surprised how many people I have met at the grocery stores. I see someone staring at the gluten-free aisle and I say hello and ask if they are gluten-free. I have met some wonderful people this way. There are many support groups for mothers available. Check your local meetup.com.

For further information about steps 1-10 please refer to *Gluten-Free Living 101: A Step by Step Guide*. For detailed personal care product information, please refer to *Is Gluten Hiding in Your Shampoo? It Was Hiding in Mine!*

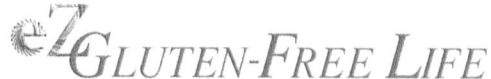

DISORDER AND DISEASE RELATED TO GLUTEN

As research improves, the array of disorders, diseases, and medical issues believed to be affected by gluten is growing. Several of the well known disorders/diseases are:

Autism (ASD) and other Behavioral Disorders are now being linked to gluten and dairy. Autism is a brain disorder that presents itself differently in different children. The disorder has a spectrum of symptoms ranging from difficulty with communication and social skill to much more extreme symptoms.

Celiac disease (CD) is also known as celiac sprue or gluten-sensitive enteropathy. It is an autoimmune disease which is genetic and therefore inherited disease. It affects people of all ages and it is believed that approximately 1 in 141 people have Celiac disease, yet most are undiagnosed. When gluten is eaten, the small intestine becomes damaged. The villi are pushed down by the gluten, creating an environment that is unable to absorb nutrients. There are over 300 registered symptoms for Celiac. The most common symptoms are diarrhea, bloating, anemia, chronic fatigue, weakness, bone pain, weight loss and muscle cramps. It was once thought that Celiac disease only affected the small intestine, but it is now known that it can causes medical issues. (Green p.2-4)

There are other disorders that can come from gluten intolerance:

Dermatitis Herpetiformis is the same disease as Celiac but the symptoms manifest themselves under the skin causing "groups of watery, itchy blisters that may resemble pimples or blisters." (gluten.net # 29.) Dermatitis herpetiformis is usually the primary symptom and the small intestinal symptoms are reduced. (gluten.net # 29.)

Autoimmune Disease: Research has begun to prove that many autoimmune diseases are triggered or affected by the consumption of gluten.

Hashimoto's is an autoimmune thyroid disorder. It is believed that when gluten is eaten the body believes it is a foreign substance and sends histamines to attack the gluten. The histamines can mistake the thyroid for gluten and attack it instead. This can occur in other organs of the body as well. (Kharrazian, p.5-8)

Gluten Ataxia is when gluten toxins affect the brain causing neurological problems such as balance issues, coordination and speech problems. (Boyd. Pg 4)

Non-Celiac Gluten Sensitivity symptoms are similar to Celiac, but unlike Celiac disease the symptoms extend past the digestive system. Symptoms include brain fog, headaches, joint pain, numbness of the arms & legs, muscle cramps, and chronic fatigue.

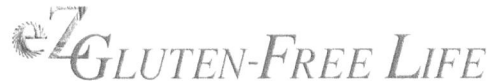

SO, WHAT IS GLUTEN ANYWAY?

Gluten has many different meanings, depending on who you are. Webster defines gluten as, "gray, sticky, nutritious substances found in wheat flour." My friend is a bread baker and to him, gluten is the substance that adds elasticity to baked goods, it helps the baked goods rise and makes the baked goods chewy. To Celiac or Hashimoto's patient, gluten is the substance that makes them feel very sick.

Gluten is the protein associated with autoimmune diseases, Celiac disease, Dermatitis Herpetiformis, Gluten Ataxia, gluten sensitivities, Hashimoto's, Autism and other disorders. The specific gluten that causes these disorders and diseases can be found in **wheat, barley, rye** (sometimes known as WBR) and possibly **oats**, (due to cross contamination) and products made with these ingredients. Dr. Peter Green, author of *Celiac Disease, A Hidden Epidemic* ,states that, "Gluten is the term for the storage protein of wheat. Wheat is approximately 10 to 15 percent protein; remainder is starch. Gluten is what remains after the starch granules are washed from the wheat flour." (Green, p. 21).

The term "gluten" has become a generic term for the specific gluten found in wheat, barley and rye which causes damage to the body, if a person is sensitive to it. There is more than one type of gluten. Corn and rice have a gluten protein that are not related to the gluten found in wheat, barley, rye and oats and are safe to eat. This book uses the word "gluten" to refer to gluten found in **wheat, barley, rye and possibly oats**. The same is usually true when recipe books, food labels, blogs, etc. use the word gluten. Gliadin is a storage protein found in **wheat**. Secalin is the storage protein found in **rye**. Hordein is the storage protein found in **barley**. These specific storage proteins are the gluten proteins that are associated with Celiac and other gluten intolerances.

You will rarely find the word gluten written in the ingredients list. Oh, if it where that simple. Wheat, barley and rye (WBR) also have genus names (see page 10) which may be used in the ingredients list. In addition, there are many forms of wheat, some which do not include the word wheat. Here is a basic list of grains and flours that contain gluten used in food sources: This information was compiled for various sources, please see reference page for details.

For the sake of this handbook GF refers to Gluten-Free which are products and items **not containing** any gluten derived from wheat, barley, rye and oats (not GF).

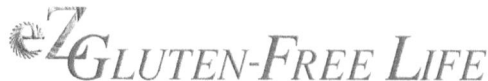

ALTERNATIVE NAMES FOR WHEAT, BARLEY, AND RYE

Barley: genus Hordeum

For more information: http://www.gramene.org/species/hordeum/barley_intro.html
Other Names for Barley

Barley Grass	Pearl Barley
Barley Hordeum Vulgare	Malt or Malt Flavoring
Barley Malt or Malt Barley	Caramel Coloring (can be made with malt barley)

Oat: genus Avena *(Celiac patients and people who have been told to avoid cross contamination need to eat gluten- free oats and follow Celiac Spruce protocol unless otherwise instructed by a physician. Please refer to this website for further information.)*
http://www.csaceliacs.info/guide_to_oats.jsp)
According to www.livingwithout.com, pure, uncontaminated oats (up to ½ cup dry oats daily) can be tolerated by most celiac patients.

Rye: genus Secale

For more information: http://www.gramene.org/species/secale/rye_intro.html

Triticale is a wheat/rye hybrid
For more information: ftp://ftp.fao.org/docrep/fao/009/y5553e/y5553e01.pdf

Wheat: genus Triticum
Other names for wheat:

Bulgur	Gliadin	Wheat Berry
Couscous	Gluten Peptides	Wheat Germ
Dinkle	Graham	Wheat Germ Oil
Durum	Kamut	Wheat Gluten
Emmer	Seitan	Wheatgrass
Faro	Semolina	Wheat Nut
Fu	Spelt	Wheat Starch

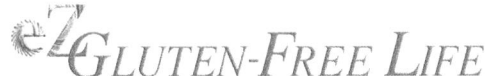

WHERE SHOULD YOU LOOK FOR GLUTEN?

Gluten can be found lurking in numerous places and many of them are unexpected. As you have begun to realize, eliminating gluten means understanding the terminology used so that you can actually read labels. In addition, it is important to know what types of products you need to be looking at. Here is a general summary of places you may find gluten.

Here is a sampling of unusual places you may find gluten. For your convenience, I have placed the name of the handbook that relates to the topic in parenthesis after the topic.

- **Alcoholic Beverages:** *(Is Gluten Hiding in Unexpected Places?)*
- **Art Supplies:** crayons, glue, finger paints, clay, play dough, & paint *(Is Gluten Hiding in Your Kid's Things?)*
- **Baked goods:** Any baked goods made with wheat, barley, rye & oats
- **Body Care Products:** deodorant, lotions, body soaps, sunscreen *(Is Gluten Hiding in Your Shampoo?)*
- **Candy** *(Is Gluten Hiding in Unexpected Places?)*
- **Cosmetics:** There are over 200 scientific names used for gluten in the processing of cosmetic and body care products. *(Is Gluten Hiding in Your Shampoo?)*
- **Dental Products:** toothpastes and oral hygiene products. *(Is Gluten Hiding in Your Shampoo?)*
- **Diapers & Training Pants:** Some brands and types contain oats. *(Is Gluten Hiding in Your Kid's Things?)*
- **Fast Food French Fries:** *(Is Gluten Hiding in Unexpected Places?)*
  - *Example:* McDonald's French Fries are coated with a beef extract made with wheat and dairy. In addition, fryers are often used for other items that contain gluten which would contaminate the oil.
- **Fast Food:** All fast food restaurants have items with gluten. *(Is Gluten Hiding in Unexpected Places?)*
- **Foods:** Foods may contain gluten, especially processed foods.
- **Hair Products:** shampoo, conditioners, hair dyes, etc. *(Is Gluten Hiding in Your Shampoo?)*
- **Household Cleaning Products:** dish soap, cleaners, laundry detergent *(Is Gluten Hiding in Unexpected Places?)*
- **Medications:** Gluten can be used in the fillers of medications. *(Is Gluten Hiding in Your Shampoo?)*
- **Nail Products:** Nail polish & other products *(Is Gluten Hiding in Your Shampoo?)*
- **Sauces:** used to cooking *(Is Gluten Hiding in Unexpected Places?)*
- **Spices:** *(Is Gluten Hiding in Unexpected Places?)*
- **Supplements:** Are regulated by the FALCPA (Food Allergen Labeling and Consumer Protection Act) that went into effect 1/1/06. If a product contains any ingredients which are derived from milk, egg, fish, crustacean shellfish, tree nuts, wheat, peanuts, and soybeans, it is clearly labeled. *(Is Gluten Hiding in Your Shampoo?)*

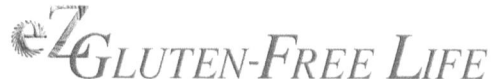

GLUTEN-FREE RESOURCES:

BOOKS on Celiac and Hashimoto's Disease

Celiac Disease, A Hidden Epidemic
Author: Dr. Peter Green and Rory Jones

Wheat Belly
Author: William Davis, M.D.

Healthier Without Wheat
Dr. Stephen Wangen

Why Do I Still Have Thyroid Symptoms? When My Lab Tests are Normal
Author: Dr. Kharrazian, DHSc, DC, MS, MNeuroSci

MAGAZINES:
1. Living Without (My favorite) www.LivingWithout.com
2. Gluten-Free Living www.glutenfreeliving.com
3. Delight gluten free www.delightglutenfree.com
4. Simply Gluten Free Magazine www.simplyglutenfreemag.com
5. CSA Lifeline
   (http://www.csaceliacs.info/and become a member to receive this
   magazine filled with current nformation)

References for page 8.
1. Boyd, Christine. "Gluten Attack: Ataxia Is gluten attacking your brain?" *Living Without Magazine*.
Feb/Mar 2011 Issue. Page 4.
2. Schneider, Lynda. "MD. Restaurant Rules." *Living Without Magazine*. June/July 2011.
3. Kharrazian, Datis DHSc, DC, MS. MNeuroSci. "Why Do I Still Have Thyroid Symptoms? When My Lab Results
Are Normal." Elephant Printing LLC; 1 edition. February 2, 2010.

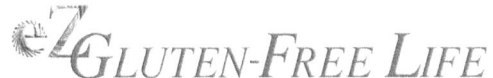

eZ GLUTEN-FREE LIFE

eZ GLUTEN-FREE LIFE WEB INFORMATION:

Web page   www.ezglutenfreelife.com
Blog   ezglutenfreelife.blogspot.com
Pinterest   http://pinterest.com/ezglutenfreelif/
FaceBook   https://www.facebook.com/EZGlutenFreeLife?ref=hl

INFORMATIONAL WEBSITES:

http://www.csaceliacs.org

http://www.csaceliacs.info/cel_kids_recipes.jsp

http://www.gfco.org/

http://www.thyroidbook.com

http://www.godairyfree.org/Food-to-Eat/Food-Label-Info/Dairy-Ingredient-List.html

RECIPES WEBSITES:

The Gluten-free Goddess is by far my favorite "go to" gluten-free with dairy free alternative recipes website.

http://glutenfreegoddess.blogspot.com

http://glutenfreegoddess.blogspot.com/2007/01/cooking-baking-gluten-free-tips-for.html

www.ohsheglows.com (vegan and often GF)

http://www.elanaspantry.com

http://glutenfreecooking.about.com/od/glutenfreecookingbasics/u/userpaths
glutenfreecooking.htm#s2

http://www.glutenfreegoddess.blogspot.com/p/how-to-go-g-free.html

http://glutenfreerecipebox.com/gluten-free-fast-food

http://www.livingwithout.com

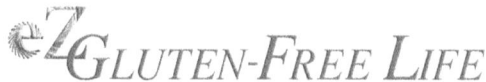

Infants & Babies: Baby Laundry Detergent	GF	GLUTEN/CC
Baby Laundry Detergent and Softener		
Amway		Undetermined
Dabble		Undetermined
Dreft	GF	
ECOS Free and Clear	GF	
		EXCEPT
Method	GF	
Ms Meyers	GF	
VERIFIED 2013		

Infants & Babies: Body Care & Hair Products	GF	GLUTEN/CC
100% Pure Cosmetics and Body Care	GF	
365 Premium Body Care	GF	
Aveeno		CC
Baby Magic	GF	
Burt's Bees		Undetermined
California Baby	GF	
Dakota Free	GF	
Dr. Bronner	GF	
VERIFIED 2013		

COMPANY INFORMATION

▲ "Gluten is not an ingredient in our detergents"

Q: Is your laundry detergent gluten-free and casein-free?

A: Yes, our laundry detergent is gluten-free and casein-free.
All of our products are gluten-free except for our Orange Plus Cleaning Towels, which contain wheat germ.

www.methodhome.com/support/faqs/

▲ "Thanks so much for taking the time to write to us and for your interest in method. Actually, all of our products are gluten free and safe for those with Celiac's disease.
We don't use wheat or gluten in any of our ingredients."

▲ "...Our products are wheat and gluten free. That being said, the equipment used to manufacture our products is not dedicated equipment, so there is a very slim chance of cross contamination. Good sterilization and separation practices are employed to avoid cross contamination."

ALWAYS READ INGREDIENTS LABELS!!!

COMPANY INFORMATION

http://www.100percentpure.com/Articles.asp?ID=146

GIG certified Whole Foods Brand

Has oat ingredients in all has products

http://www.babymagic.com/q&a

www.burtsbees.com

http://www.californiababy.com/

https://dakotafree.com/Category.asp?Category_Id=5

All products are GF

ALWAYS READ INGREDIENTS LABELS!!!

Infants & Babies: Body Care & Hair Products	GF	GLUTEN/CC
Earth Mama Angel Baby Organics	GF	
Eco	GF	
Exederm	GF	
Hugo Naturals	GF	
Jason		Read Labels
Kissmyface		
Kids Natural Suncreen Block spf 30	GF	
Little Twig	GF	
Method	GF	
Monkey Sea Monkey Doo	GF	
Neutrogena		Undetermined
Nourish	GF	
NuSkin	GF	
		EXCEPT
NuSkin		
Organique by Himalaya Herbals		Read Info
Green Labels are GF	GF	
Rainbow Research	GF	
VERIFIED 2013		

COMPANY INFORMATION

▲ http://www.earthmamaangelbaby.com

All products are GF except:

Angel Baby Lotion and Earth Mama Body Butter

www.ecologicalskin.com (dedicated facility)

No Gluten Added

http://hugonaturals.com/about-our-products

Read labels some of the products do contain wheat

▲ "Our Plant-based formulations come from a variety of sources and combinations of derivatives and are not screened for traces of specific allergens. We cannot guarantee that our products are gluten-free."

http://www.kissmyface.com/product/item/121

Many products are GF read labels

www.littletwig.com

▲ http://methodhome.com/support/faqs/

"Thanks so much for taking the time to write to us and for your interest in method. Actually, all of our products are gluten free and safe for those with Celiac's disease. We don't use wheat or gluten in any of our ingredients."

monkeyseamonkeydoo.com (dedicated facility)

Line too extensive to give details- email about specific products.

www.nourishUSDA.com (dedicated facility)

▲ All Products GF Except:

AHA Facial Peel (oat kernel extract)

Balancing Shampoo (wheat)

Epoch Baby Hibiscus (oat kernel extract)

Face Lift Activator, Sensitive skin (wheat)

Face Lift Powder, Sensitive skin (wheat)

Face Lift Powder with Activator, Sensitive skin (wheat)

Moisturizing Shampoo (wheat)

StylinGel (wheat)

▲ All gluten free products labeled with green label

Full line of body & hair care for children

ALWAYS READ INGREDIENTS LABELS!!!

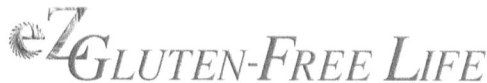

Infants & Babies: Body Care & Hair Products	GF	GLUTEN/CC
Seventh Generation Baby Line	GF	
Shampoo & Wash		
Lotions:		
Diaper Cream		
Suncreen		
Baby Wipes		
Susan Brown's Baby		Read Labels
Weleda		GLUTEN
VERIFIED 2013		

Infants & Babies: Diapers	GF	GLUTEN/CC
Babies R Us Line of Baby Products		Undetermined
gDiapers	GF	
Huggies (see below Kimberly Clark)		
Huggies®		**EXCEPT**
Huggies® Diapers	GF	
Pull Ups	GF	
Good Nites	GF	
Little Swimmers	GF	
Pampers	GF	
Seventh Generation	GF	
Diapers used for Day		**EXCEPT**
VERIFIED 2013		

COMPANY INFORMATION

▲ Shampoo & Wash, Bubble Bath, Lotion. Diaper Cream, Sunscreen, Baby Wipes

▲ http://www.susanbrownsbaby.com/
Some products contain oats- read labels

▲ http://usa.weleda.com/footer/faq.aspx
"As a natural component of wheat, it is found in some of the ingredients we use in our products. Many of our skin care products include small quantities of organic alcohol derived from organic wheat. A few products are also formulated with Triticum Vulgare (Wheat Germ) Oil. We cannot guarantee that these ingredients are entirely free of all traces of gluten."

ALWAYS READ INGREDIENTS LABELS!!!

COMPANY INFORMATION

Unable to answer my questions

No Gluten added

Kimberly-Clark consumer products do not contain:

Huggies®Soft Skin Products - contain oats

No Gluten added

http://seventhgeneration.custhelp.com/app/answers/list

▲ Trainings Pants & Overnight Diapers
"Our Free and Clear diapers and wipes are gluten free. However, our training pants and overnight diapers use a wheat based ingredient for the absorbent core of the diapers."

ALWAYS READ INGREDIENTS LABELS!!!

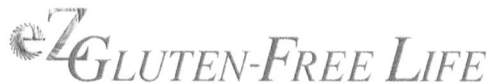

Infants & Babies: Diaper Rash Cream	GF	GLUTEN/CC
A&D lotion		Undetermined
Aquaphor		Undetermined
Aveeno		Contains Oats
California Baby	GF	
Desitin		Undetermined
MonkeySeaMonkeyDoo Diaper Balm)	GF	
Triple Paste		Contains Oats
VERIFIED 2013		

Infants & Babies: Baby Wipes	GF	GLUTEN/CC
Babies R Us		Undetermined
Baby Genics		Undetermined
California Baby	GF	
Disney Baby		Undetermined
Especially for Kids		Undetermined
Fischer Price		Undetermined
gDiapers	GF	
Pampers	GF	
Wet Ones (Wipes)		Undetermined
VERIFIED 2013		

COMPANY INFORMATION

http://www.myadbaby.com/

http://www.aquaphorhealing.com/#/main?ovr=faq

Has oat ingredients in all has products

http://www.californiababy.com/

http://www.desitin.com/frequently-asked-questions

http://monkeyseamonkeydoo.com/

http://www.triplepaste.com/frequently-asked-questions/

Has oats in it but no wheat, barley and rye

ALWAYS READ INGREDIENTS LABELS!!!

COMPANY INFORMATION

Could not answer my questions. Read Labels

Unable to confirm either way.

http://www.californiababy.com/

Unknown - read labels

Unknown - read labels

Unable to confirm either way.

No Gluten added

No Gluten added

▲ I received the same response over the phone.

We understand your concern about ensuring the products you are using do not contain gluten. With regard to our line of sun care products, although we do not use wheat protein or wheat derived oils in our product formulations, we cannot certify that our facilities are gluten-free. In addition, the plant origin of some ingredients may vary, making Gluten Free Certification difficult. We regret we are not able to suggest a product that meets your needs at this time. For specific information on this ingredient as well as other sun care and cosmetic product ingredients, please visit www.cosmeticsinfo.org.

ALWAYS READ INGREDIENTS LABELS!!!

Infants & Babies: Lotions	GF	GLUTEN/CC
Aveeno		Contains Oats
Burt's Bees		Undetermined
Baby Genics		Undetermined
Baby Magic	GF	
Babies R Us		Undetermined
California Baby	GF	
Earth's Best -Organic		Read Info
(owned by Hain Celestrial)		
These are the symbols you will see on their products if they are 100% GF		
Earth Mama Angel Baby Organics	GF	
		EXCEPT
EO	GF	
California Baby	GF	
Coppertone	GF	

OUR GLUTEN-FREE
GUARANTEE
You can count on us!

Gluten
Free

Certified
(GF)
Gluten-Free

VERIFIED 2013

COMPANY INFORMATION

www.aveeno.com

www.burtsbees.com

Unable to confirm either way.

http://www.babymagic.com/q&a

Could not answer my questions. Read Labels

http://www.californiababy.com/

▲ http://www.earthsbest.com/node/17

Website suggests reading labels of individual items.

Many of there products are made without gluten.

http://www.glutenfreechoices.com/

This group understands GF and is a supporter.

Please see http://www.glutenfreechoices.com/

"Consumer health and safety is our number one concern. We do not have lists of products that are specifically considered to be gluten free. Reading the label is the best way to check for the presence of ingredients which contain gluten.If gluten is a major ingredient, it will be specified in the ingredient list. For consumers concerned about the presence of trace amounts of gluten, we suggest avoiding products that include natural flavors or spices."

http://www.earthmamaangelbaby.com

Angel Baby Lotion and Earth Mama Body Butter

GIG certified

http://www.californiababy.com/

▲ Water Babies Pure & Simple

1-866-288-3330 called 3/12

Coppertone is in the process of testing all their products and updating the website to include gluten-free information. They say all their product are gluten-free.

ALWAYS READ INGREDIENTS LABELS!!!

e Z *GLUTEN-FREE LIFE*

Kid's: Art	GF	GLUTEN/CC
Crayons		
Crayola		
All Crayola	GF	Read Info
Colorations		
Large Crayons	GF	
Colored Pencils		
Crayola		
All Crayola	GF	Read Info
Finger Paints		
Crayola		
All Crayola Finger Paints	GF	
Elmer's		GLUTEN
Glue		
Aleene's		
Original Tacky Glue	GF	
Crafty Dab		
School & Craft White Glue	GF	
Clear School Glue	GF	
Glue Continuation		
Coloration		
Clear Glue Gun Refill	GF	
Confetti Glitter Glue	GF	
Glitter Glue	GF	
Purple Washable Glue Sticks	GF	
Rainbow Glitter Glue	GF	
Tacky Glue Pen	GF	
Washable Premium GlueSticks	GF	
Washable School Glue	GF	
All Elmer's Glue	GF	
Mod Podge	GF	
Glue with latex		
Rubber Cement	GF	

VERIFIED 2013

COMPANY INFORMATION

▲ *Crayola email response is attached so that you can read it and decided for yourself.*

Free of gluten, dairy/casein, egg, latex, peanut/tree nut & soy (discountschoolsupplies.com)

Free of gluten, dairy/casein, egg, latex, peanut/tree nut & soy (discountschoolsupplies.com)

Free of gluten, dairy/casein, egg, latex, peanut/tree nut & soy (discountschoolsupplies.com)

(Check all finger paints before using)

Free of gluten, dairy/casein, egg, latex, peanut/tree nut & soy (discountschoolsupplies.com)

Elmer's Finger Paints contains wheat and oat products.

▲ *ELMER'S FINGER PAINTS ARE NOT GLUTEN FREE!*

Wheat gluten is sometimes used to make glue for envelopes, stamps etc.

Free of gluten, dairy/casein, egg, latex, peanut/tree nut & soy (discountschoolsupplies.com)

Free of gluten, dairy/casein, egg, latex, peanut/tree nut & soy (discountschoolsupplies.com)

Free of gluten, dairy/casein, egg, latex, peanut/tree nut & soy (discountschoolsupplies.com)

Wheat gluten is sometimes used to make glue for envelopes, stamps etc.

Free of gluten, dairy/casein, egg, latex, peanut/tree nut & soy (discountschoolsupplies.com)

Free of gluten, dairy/casein, egg, latex, peanut/tree nut & soy (discountschoolsupplies.com)

Free of gluten, dairy/casein, egg, latex, peanut/tree nut & soy (discountschoolsupplies.com)

Free of gluten, dairy/casein, egg, latex, peanut/tree nut & soy (discountschoolsupplies.com)

Free of gluten, dairy/casein, egg, latex, peanut/tree nut & soy (discountschoolsupplies.com)

Free of gluten, dairy/casein, egg, latex, peanut/tree nut & soy (discountschoolsupplies.com)

Free of gluten, dairy/casein, egg, latex, peanut/tree nut & soy (discountschoolsupplies.com)

Elmer's reported that all their products are gluten free except Elmer's Finger Paint

Free of gluten, dairy/casein, egg, latex, peanut/tree nut & soy (discountschoolsupplies.com)

Free of dairy/casein, egg, peanut/tree nut & soy (discountschoolsupplies.com)

ALWAYS READ INGREDIENTS LABELS!!!

Kid's: Art	GF	GLUTEN/CC
Ink Pads		
Colorations		
Classic Colors &Candy Colors	GF	
Jumbo Washable Stamp Pads		
Metallic Washable Stamp Pads	GF	
Stamper Perfect Washable	GF	
Stamp Pads		
Markers		
Crayola		
All Crayola	GF	
Colorations		
Super Washable Classic Marker	GF	
Washable Cubby Markers	GF	
Dot-A-Dot Marker Set	GF	
Colorations		
Dry Erase Bullet Tip Markers	GF	
Fabric Markers	GF	
Modeling Clay		
Aroma-dough	GF	
Crayola		
Model Magic	GF	
Modeling Clay		
Air-Dry Clay		
Model Magic Fusion		
Discount School		
Non-Hardening Model Clay	GF	
Supply		
Super Light-Weight Air-Dry Putty	GF	
Moist Red Modeling Clay	GF	

VERIFIED 2013

COMPANY INFORMATION

Free of dairy/casein, egg, peanut/tree nut & soy (discountschoolsupplies.com)

Free of dairy/cas Free of dairy/casein, egg, peanut/tree nut & soy (discountschoolsupplies.com)

Free of gluten, dairy/casein, egg, latex, peanut/tree nut & soy (discountschoolsupplies.com)

Free of gluten, dairy/casein, egg, latex, peanut/tree nut & soy (discountschoolsupplies.com)
Free of gluten, dairy/casein, egg, latex, peanut/tree nut & soy (discountschoolsupplies.com)
Free of gluten, dairy/casein, egg, latex, peanut/tree nut & soy (discountschoolsupplies.com)

Free of gluten, dairy/casein, egg, latex, peanut/tree nut & soy (discountschoolsupplies.com)
Free of gluten, dairy/casein, egg, latex, peanut/tree nut & soy (discountschoolsupplies.com)

Free of dairy/casein, egg, peanut/tree nut & soy (discountschoolsupplies.com)
As per the email attached these products are wheat free, dairy/casien, egg, latex, peanut/tree nut, legumes & soy (discountschoolsupplies.com)

Free of gluten, dairy/casien, egg, latex, peanut/tree nut & soy (discountschoolsupplies.com)

Free of gluten, dairy/casien, egg, latex, peanut/tree nut & soy (discountschoolsupplies.com)
Free of gluten, dairy/casien, egg, latex, peanut/tree nut & soy (discountschoolsupplies.com)

ALWAYS READ INGREDIENTS LABELS!!!

Kid's: Art	GF	GLUTEN/CC
Play Dough		
FOR FAMILY FUN, SEE RECIPES BELOW.		
Aroma-dough	GF	
Mama K's		
Play Clay	GF	
Alex's Toys		GLUTEN
Crayola		GLUTEN
Play Doh		GLUTEN
Rose Arts		GLUTEN

Gluten-Free Play Dough Recipes:

Gluten-Free Play Dough Recipe: http://www.csaceliacs.info/cel_kids_recipes.jsp

Play Dough Ingredients:

    $1/2$ cup rice flour
    $1/2$ cup cornstarch
    $1/2$ cup salt
    2 teaspoons cream of tartar
    1 cup water
    1 teaspoon cooking oil
    Food coloring, if desired

Directions:
    1. Mix all ingredients together.
    2. Cook and stir on low heat for 3 minutes or until it forms a ball.
    3. Cool completely before storing in a sealable plastic bag.

VERIFIED 2013

COMPANY INFORMATION

Free of dairy/casein, egg, peanut/tree nut & soy (discountschoolsupplies.com)
Uses all natural products, http://www.mama-ks.com/

Alex's Toys: "Our dough contains gluten that comes from wheat. It is a required element that determines the elasticity."
▲ *CRAYOLA DOUGH IS NOT GLUTEN FREE*
SEE CRAYOLA EMAIL RESPONSE ATTACHED.
▲ *CRAYOLA DOUGH IS NOT GLUTEN FREE*

Rose Arts: Mega Dough and Fun Dough have GLUTEN. All other products are GF.

Living Without Magazine's Dec/Jan 2012 issue written by Madalene Rhyand

Play Clay Ingredients: (makes 2 pounds)
　1 cup potato starch or corn starch
　2 cups baking soda
　1 cup cold water
　1 tablespoon vegetable oil of choice
　2-3 drops of food color (optional)

Directions:
　1. Mix together potato starch and baking soda and pour in saucepan.
　2. Mix water and oil in small bowl. Add food coloring, if using.
　3. Heat saucepan and pour water and oil, stirring constantly about 3 minutes or until clay holds together in a ball. (Small lumps will appear and then clay will hold together.)
　4. Turn off heat. Spoon clay onto parchment paper and let cool slightly.
　5. Roll clay in parchment paper forming a cylinder and let cool completely. Knead a little before using.

ALWAYS READ INGREDIENTS LABELS!!!

Kid's: Art	GF	GLUTEN/CC
Paint		
BioColor Paints	GF	
Colorations		
Fabric Paints	GF	
Finger Paints	GF	
Liquid Watercolor Paint	GF	
No-Drip Foam Paint	GF	
Simply Washable Tempura Paint	GF	
Washable Glitter Paint	GF	
Crayola		
Finger Paint	GF	
Paint		
Elmer's		
3D Washable Paint Pens:	GF	
Classic Colors	GF	
Bold Colors	GF	
Bright Colors	GF	
Finger Paints		
Crayola		
All Finger Paints	GF	
Elmer's		GLUTEN
Paper Mache		
AMACO		
Rice Paste Powder	GF	
BUY GF ART SUPPLIES		
ONLINE		
ONLINE		
ONLINE		
VERIFIED 2013		

COMPANY INFORMATION

Free of gluten, dairy/casien, egg, latex, peanut/tree nut & soy (discountschoolsupplies.com)

Free of gluten, dairy/casien, egg, latex, peanut/tree nut & soy (discountschoolsupplies.com)
Free of gluten, dairy/casien, egg, latex, peanut/tree nut & soy (discountschoolsupplies.com)
Free of gluten, dairy/casien, egg, latex, peanut/tree nut & soy (discountschoolsupplies.com)
Free of gluten, dairy/casien, egg, latex, peanut/tree nut & soy (discountschoolsupplies.com)
Free of gluten, dairy/casien, egg, latex, peanut/tree nut & soy (discountschoolsupplies.com)
Free of gluten, dairy/casien, egg, latex, peanut/tree nut & soy (discountschoolsupplies.com)

Free of gluten, dairy/casien, egg, latex, peanut/tree nut & soy & D&C Red Dye #40

Free of gluten, dairy/casein, egg, latex, peanut/tree nut & soy (discountschoolsupplies.com)

Elmer's Finger Paints contains wheat and oat products.
Check all finger paints before using them.

http://www.amaco.com/product-search-results/?qProd=Papier+Mache&x=0&y=0

Places to purchase Gluten-Free art products online.
Discountschoolsupply.com (GF art materials such as markers, crayons, glue, and paints.)
Amazon.com
Aroma-dough.com

ALWAYS READ INGREDIENTS LABELS!!!

Kid's: Body Care and Hair Products	GF	GLUTEN/CC
100% Pure Cosmetics and Body Care	GF	
365 Premium Body Care	GF	
Aubrey		Read Labels
Aveeno		CC
Baby Magic	GF	
Burt's Bees		Undetermined
California Baby	GF	
Dakota Free	GF	
Dr. Bronner	GF	
Earth Mama Angel Baby Organics	GF	
Eco	GF	
Exederm	GF	
Hugo Naturals	GF	
Jason's		Read Info
Johnson & Johnson		Read Info
Kissmyface:		
Kid's Self Foaming Hand Soaps	GF	
Kid's Lip Balm	GF	
Kid's Whale Soap	GF	
Kid's Natural Mineral Sun Screen SPF 30	GF	
Kid's Bubble Wash	GF	
Kid's Toothpaste	GF	
Kid's Sun Sticks	GF	
Little Twig	GF	
L'Oreal		CC
VERIFIED 2013		

COMPANY INFORMATION

http://www.100percentpure.com/Articles.asp? ID=146

GIG certified Whole Foods Brand

www.aubrey.com There is Gluten in many of the products

▲ Has oat ingredients in all has products

http://www.babymagic.com/q&a

www.burtsbees.com

http://www.californiababy.com/

https://dakotafree.com/Category.asp?Category_Id=5

ALL PRODUCTS ARE GF

http://www.earthmamaangelbaby.com

All products are GF except:

▲ Angel Baby Lotion and Earth Mama Body Butter

www.ecologicalskin.com (dedicated facility)

No Gluten Added

http://hugonaturals.com/about-our-products

▲ "Our Plant-based formulations come from a variety of sources and combinations of derivatives and are not screened for traces of specific allergens. We cannot guarantee that our products are gluten-free."

Extra Gentle Kids Shampoo has GLUTEN

▲ Though many of Johnson & Johnson's products do not contain gluten, the company can not comment on cross contaminaition due to the extensive line.

http://www.kissmyface.com/product/item/121

www.littletwig.com

www.lorealparisusa.com

ALWAYS READ INGREDIENTS LABELS!!!

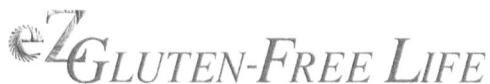

Kid's: Body Care and Hair Products	GF	GLUTEN/CC
Method	GF	
Monkey Sea Monkey Doo	GF	
Neutrogena		Undetermined
Nourish	GF	
NuSkin	GF	
		EXCEPT
Organique by Himalaya Herbals		Read Labels
Rainbow Research	GF	
Sauve		**GLUTEN/CC**
Seventh Generation Baby Line	GF	
Susan Brown's Baby		Read Labels
Weleda		**GLUTEN**
VERIFIED 2013		

COMPANY INFORMATION

http://methodhome.com/support/faqs/
▲ "Thanks so much for taking the time to write to us and for your interest in method. Actually, all of our products are gluten free and safe for those with Celiac's disease. We don't use wheat or gluten in any of our ingredients."

monkeyseamonkeydoo.com (dedicated facility)
Line too extensive to give details- email about specific products.

www.nourishUSDA.com (dedicated facility)
▲ All Products GF Except:
AHA Facial Peel (oat kernel extract)
Balancing Shampoo (wheat)
Epoch Baby Hibiscus (oat kernel extract)
Face Lift Activator, Sensitive skin (wheat)
Face Lift Powder, Sensitive skin (wheat)
Face Lift Powder with Activator, Sensitive skin (wheat)
Moisturizing Shampoo (wheat)
StylinGel (wheat)
▲ All gluten free products labeled with green label.

Organic baby & kids line of GF products
Body washes, shampoos, conditioners, detanglers

▲ Shampoo & Wash, Bubble Bath, lotion. Diaper cream, sunscreen, Baby wipes
http://www.susanbrownsbaby.com/
▲ Some products contain oats- read labels

http://usa.weleda.com/footer/faq.aspx
▲ "As a natural component of wheat, it is found in some of the ingredients we use in our products. Many of our skin care products include small quantities of organic alcohol derived from organic wheat. A few products are also formulated with Triticum Vulgare (Wheat Germ) Oil. We cannot guarantee that these ingredients are entirely free of all traces of gluten."

ALWAYS READ INGREDIENTS LABELS!!!

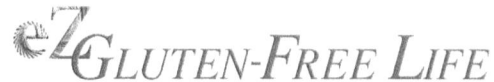

Kid's: Lotion	GF	GLUTEN/CC
Aveeno		CC
Baby Magic	GF	
Babies R Us		Undetermined
Burt's Bees		Undetermined
California Baby	GF	
Earth Mama Angel Baby Organics	GF	
Earth's Best(owned by Hain Celestrial)		Read Info

These are the symbols you will see on
their products if they are 100% GF

OUR GLUTEN-FREE
GUARANTEE
You can count on us!

Gluten Free / Certified GF Gluten-Free

VERIFIED 2013

COMPANY INFORMATION

▲ Has oat ingredients in all has products
http://www.babymagic.com/q&a
▲ Could not answer my questions. Read Labels
www.burtsbees.com
http://www.californiababy.com/
http://www.earthmamaangelbaby.com
All products are GF except
Angel Baby Lotion and Earth Mama Body Butter
▲ http://www.earthsbest.com/node/17

Website suggests reading labels of individual items.
Many of there products are made without gluten
http://www.glutenfreechoices.com/
Hain-Celestrials: Owns Earths Baby
This group understands GF and is a supporter. Please see
http://www.glutenfreechoices.com/
Consumer health and safety is our number one concern.
We do not have lists of products that are specifically considered to be gluten free.
Reading the label is the best way to check for the presence of ingredients which
contain gluten. If gluten is a major ingredient, it will be specified in the ingredient list.
For consumers concerned about the presence of trace amounts of gluten, we suggest
avoiding products that include natural flavors or spices.

ALWAYS READ INGREDIENTS LABELS!!!

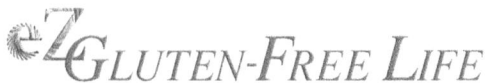

Kid's: Sunscreen	GF	GLUTEN/CC
IMPORTANT:		
Alba Botanica		Undetermined
All Terrain	GF	
Arbonne	GF	
Aveeno		Contains Oats
Baby Blanket		
Badger	GF	Read Info
Banana Boat		Contact Company
Burt's Bees		Contact Company
California Baby	GF	
Coppertone	GF	
Water Babies& Kids Pure & Simple	GF	
UltraGuard SPF 30	GF	
Solacane	GF	
VERIFIED 2013		

COMPANY INFORMATION

According to the FDA children under 6 months old should not have sunscreen put on them.

http://www.fda.gov/ForConsumers/ConsumerUpdates/ucm309136.htm

www.albabotanica.com

▲ "Our plant-based formulations come from a variety of sources and combinations of derivatives and are not screened for traces of specific allergens. We cannot guarantee that our products are gluten-free."

www.allterrain.com

www.arbonne.com

www.aveeno.com

http://www.babyblanketsuncare.com/thanks.htm

http://www.badgerbalm.com/t-faq.aspx

▲ I have allergies to Peanuts and Gluten. Are Badger Products safe for me to use?
"Badger products contain no peanuts, peanut oils, wheat or gluten. However, the facility that fills our lip balms also uses wheat amino acids and wheat protein, so there is the possibility of cross-contamination. Our facility is not certified as "gluten free", but uses no wheat or gluten containing ingredients."

▲ "We understand your concern about ensuring the products you are using do not contain gluten. With regard to our line of sun care products, although we do not use wheat protein or wheat derived oils in our product formulations, we cannot certify that our facilities are gluten free.
In addition, the plant origin of some ingredients may vary, making Gluten Free Certification difficult. We regret we are not able to suggest a product that meets your needs at this time.
For specific information on this ingredient as well as other sun care and cosmetic product ingredients, please visit www.cosmeticsinfo.org."

www.burtsbees.com

http://www.californiababy.com/

▲ 1-866-288-3330

▲ Coppertone is in the process of testing all their products and updating the website to include gluten-free information. They say all their product are gluten-free.

ALWAYS READ INGREDIENTS LABELS!!!

GLUTEN-FREE LIFE

Kid's: Sunscreen	GF	GLUTEN/CC
Dakota Free	GF	
Desert Essences Organics	GF	
Earth's Best Baby Care		Contains Oats
Eco	GF	
Hawaiian Tropic		Contact Company
Johnson and Johnson		Undetermined
Kissmyface:		
Cell Mate Facial Crème & Suncreen	GF	
Face Factor (SP 30, SPF 50)	GF	
Hot Spotss SPF 30	GF	
Kids Sun Stick SPF 30	GF	
Sport Spray SPF 50	GF	
Sun Spray (Lotion SPF 30, Oil SPF 30)	GF	
Maui Babe		Undetermined
Neutrogena		Contact Company
Sunology		Contact Company
VERIFIED 2013		

COMPANY INFORMATION

https://dakotafree.com/Category.asp?Category_Id=5

www.ecologicalskin.com (dedicated facility)

▲ "We understand your concern about ensuring the products you are using do not contain gluten. With regard to our line of sun care products, although we do not use wheat protein or wheat derived oils in our product formulations, we cannot certify that our facilities are gluten free.
In addition, the plant origin of some ingredients may vary, making Gluten Free Certification difficult. We regret we are not able to suggest a product that meets your needs at this time.
For specific information on this ingredient as well as other sun care and cosmetic product ingredients, please visit www.cosmeticsinfo.org."

▲ While we perform comprehensive testing on the more common ingredients that may provide an allergic reaction such as gluten, nuts etc., unfortunately, it is impossible to test for every ingredient and we cannot guarantee that our products are gluten-free, since the source of an ingredient may change from time to time. Some of the ingredients in the product may have been purchased by us from outside distributors and we cannot say with absolute certainty that cross contamination with this ingredient did not occur at their facilities.

www.kissmyface.com

http://www.mauibabe.com/

Line too extensive to give details- email about specific products

www.sunology.com

ALWAYS READ INGREDIENTS LABELS!!!

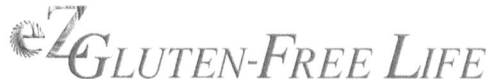

Creative Ideas to Help Children Adjust!

How do you get your children to "buy" into a healthy eating program?

1. Your Attitude: It starts with you: Be positive
2. Be a Good Role Model
3. Do not let your child see you sweat over their food issues.
4. Everyone has the right to feel safe at home! Make your home a safe zone.
5. Empower your child with knowledge and a sense of independence
    - Educate them on food and the reasons they need to eat a certain way.
    A. Role play with your child. (See next page)
    B. Play food games with them. (See page 44)
    C. Read age appropriate books together about foods, gardening, cooking etc.
6. Do not allow their food issues to define who they are. They are so much more than their food issues.
7. Always have healthy snacks available for them at home, school and when they are away from home.
8. Keep dialogues going. Make it fun and light. (See Ideas)
9. Allow your children to be a part of the menu planning, grocery shopping and cooking.
10. Set aside one day a week, so that you can prepare snacks, meals and treats for the week. Children will enjoy the ritual and you will have foods prepared when needed.
11. Take their favorite foods and find healthy alternatives. Have them be a part of the recipe experiments.
12. Eat dinner at the table, as often as possible. Shut off the TV, cell phones, and computers during this time. This eating ritual promotes conversation, family time, and a sense of belonging.

Remember you cannot always be with your child, so preparing them is essential.

Role Playing

Depending on your child's age, role playing can be a very successful tool in preparing them for various scenarios they may encounter in the outside world.

   A. Role playing with your child
- Play restaurant:
  - Teach them how to order when you are at a restaurant
  - Collect menus from some of your regular restaurants
  - Review the menu together and discuss the best choices
  - Set the table as if it is a restaurant
  - Take turns being the server and the customer. (Have a note pad for the server to write down the order.)
  - Act out possible misunderstandings
  - Giggle and laugh to make this fun
  - Act out issues that may come up in school such as; a birthday party or field trip. Role play the different roles, so your children are comfortable speaking up for themselves.
  - Role play possible scenarios they may encounter at friends homes.

   B. Play food games with them. (See page 44)

   C. Read age appropriate books together about foods, gardening, cooking, etc.

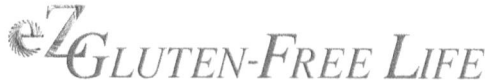

Creative Ideas to Help Children Adjust! (continued)

Food Games

The internet has many food games you can access. Always check them out before allowing your child to use them.

A. PBS: pbs.org has articles, internet games and ideas about healthy eating. http://pbskids.org/games/healthyeating.html

B. http://www.nutritionexplorations.org/kids.php

C. http://www.foodafactoflife.org.uk/QuickLinks.aspx?contentType=2

D. http://www.familylearning.org.uk/balanced_diet.html

Games you can purchase:

E. http://www.crunchacolor.com/products/crunch-a-color

F. http://www.woodlands-junior.kent.sch.uk/revision/science/living/humanbody.html

Children's Books

Amazon, Barnes & Noble's, etc have children's books and videos about healthy eating.

Here are a couple:

Eat a Rainbow: Healthy Foods (Move and Get Healthy!) [Library Binding] by Susan Temple Kesselring

Kids' Fun and Healthy Cookbook by Nicola Graim

Cooking and baking with your child

Making your child a part of the cooking process gives them a chance to "own" the food. Depending on your child's ability to focus, plan out a menu and decide which jobs they can successfully do. Do not expect them to help with the whole meal though some children will be able to.

- Make it fun
- Set up a safe work area that is size appropriate for your child (low tables or a step stool)
- Prepare ahead of time, so you can focus on the children
- Remind them of the rules of the kitchen (sharp knives, hot stove etc.)
- Have age appropriate utensils (young children can use a safe knife such as a BPA free plastic knife)
- If your child reads, they can help read the directions

Cooking and baking with your child (continued)

- Measuring the ingredients is a great way for a child to visualize some of the math concepts they are learning
- This is a great time to introduce new foods. (Instead of banana bread you could make carrot bread or zucchini bread. Instead of rice you could substitute quinoa)
- Enjoy the food together

Conversations

A. Convert the verbal game, Animal, Vegetable, and Mineral into a food game.
- I am thinking of healthy foods
- I am thinking of unhealthy foods
- I am thinking of occasional treats, etc.

Ask Questions:
- Is it a fruit, veggie or protein?
- Is it considered a real food or processed food?
- Does it have more than 5 ingredients?

B. Change up I Spy
- While you're in the grocery store you can play I Spy with food. I spy a fruit. I spy a processed food. I spy a junk food. I spy a food that can be eaten occasionally, etc.

Foods: Formula & Baby Food Companies	GF	GLUTEN/CC
Baby's Only by Nature's Only	GF	
Beech Nut		Undetermined
Earth's Best - Organic (owned by Hain Celestrial)		Read Info
Enfamil	GF	
Gerber		Undetermined
HappyFamily	GF	
Healthy Time Baby - Organic		
All jarred foods	GF	
		EXCEPT
Pediasure	GF	
Similac®	GF	

These are the symbols you will see on their products if they are 100% GF

OUR GLUTEN-FREE
GUARANTEE
You can count on us!

(Gluten Free) (GF) Certified Gluten-Free

VERIFIED 2013

COMPANY INFORMATION

▲ "Thank you for your inquiry and interest in our products.
Baby's Only Organic® formulas (this includes Baby's Only Organic® Dairy, Dairy with DHA & ARA, Lactose Free and Soy formulas) and PediaSmart® complete organic nutrition beverages are all gluten-free and can be used for gluten sensitivities, gluten enteropathies, and celiac disease. The Vitamin E used in these products is sourced from vegetable oils, not wheat and is gluten free."

Read all labels -Beware of cross contamination

▲ http://www.earthsbest.com/node/17
Website suggests reading labels of individual items.
Many of there products are made without gluten.
http://www.glutenfreechoices.com/
This group understands GF and is a supporter. Please see
http://www.glutenfreechoices.com/
"Consumer health and safety is our number one concern. We do not have lists of products that are specifically considered to be gluten free. Reading the label is the best way to check for the presence of ingredients which contain gluten.If gluten is a major ingredient, it will be specified in the ingredient list. For consumers concerned about the presence of trace amounts of gluten, we suggest avoiding products that include natural flavors or spices."

"All Mead Johnson infant formulas and pediatric products are gluten-free."

Read all labels -Beware of cross contamination

Baby Foods & Tots foods

"Brown Rice Cereal has no added gluten" They do have other cereals that have gluten and are manufactured in the same facility."

http://pediasure.com/faq

▲ All Gluten Free
"Thank you for contacting the Similac® StrongMoms® program. All Similac® infant formulas, including Similac Advance®, Similac Sensitive Similac Soy Isomil®, Similac Advance Organic, Similac Expert Care™ Alimentum®, Similac Expert Care NeoSure®, Similac Expert Care for Diarrhea, Similac Go & Grow™, and Similac For Spit-Up, are gluten-free and suitable for children with Celiac Disease or gluten sensitivity."

ALWAYS READ INGREDIENTS LABELS!!!

Foods: Toddler Food	GF	GLUTEN/CC
Beech Nut		Undetermined
Gerber		Undetermined
Earth's Best:		Read Info
(owned by Hain Celestrial)		

These are the symbols you will see on their products if they are 100% GF

OUR GLUTEN-FREE
GUARANTEE
You can count on us!

Gluten Free / Certified GF Gluten-Free

	GF	GLUTEN/CC
Happy Baby		Read Info
HAPPY**BABY** frozen meals	GF	**EXCEPT**
HAPPY**BITES** Chicken Bites	GF	
Brown Rice Cereal	GF	
HappyFamily	GF	
Healthy Time Baby		
All Jarred Foods	GF	
Brown Rice Cereal		Read Info
Teething Bisquits		
Belle Baby's	GF	
Hot Kid Baby Mum-mum	GF	
VERIFIED 2013		

COMPANY INFORMATION

Read all labels -Beware of cross contamination
Read all labels -Beware of cross contamination
http://www.earthsbest.com/node/17
Website suggests reading labels of individual items.
Many of their products are made without gluten

http://www.glutenfreechoices.com/
Hain-Celestrials: Owns Earths Baby
This group understands GF and is a supporter. Please see
http://www.glutenfreechoices.com/
Consumer health and safety is our number one concern. We do not have lists of products that are specifically considered to be gluten free. Reading the label is the best way to check for the presence of ingredients which contain gluten. If gluten is a major ingredient, it will be specified in the ingredient list. For consumers concerned about the presence of trace amounts of gluten, we suggest avoiding products that include natural flavors or spices.
http://www.happybabyfood.com/allergen-free-information
See website for all allergen information
With the exception of *Regular Prunes,*

Baby Foods & Tots Foods.
http://www.healthytimes.com/

▲ "Brown Rice Cereal has no added gluten" They do have other cereals that have gluten and are manufactured in the same facility."

PLEASE remember Wheat Free is NOT Gluten-Free.
These are the only 2 gluten-free companies I could confirm.
http://www.bellesbiscuits.com/
www.amazon.com

ALWAYS READ INGREDIENTS LABELS!!!

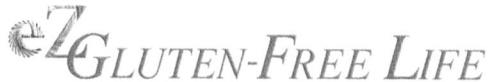

Breakfast and Lunch Menu Ideas for Kids

These are just a few suggestions to get you started.

School Lunches

1. Author & blogger Connie Sarros has some great school lunch ideas for children. "Fun Gluten-free School Lunches" by Connie Sarros http://www.avoidingmilkprotein.com/Fun.htm

2. Website for Connie Sarros recipe book for meal for kids http://glutenfreehelp.info/allergies/wheat-free-gluten-free-cookbook-for-kids-and-busy-adults-by-connie-sarros/

3. Laptop Lunches: "Laptop Lunches® bento-ware is designed to help you pack nutritious, eco-friendly lunches for school, work, travel, play or take out. Our stylish, eco-friendly lunch boxes are reusable, recyclable, long lasting, and dishwasher safe. They contain NO phthalates, bisphenol A (BPA), PVC, or lead." This website has menu ideas, recipes, newsletters etc., http://www.laptoplunches.com/safe-lunchboxes/

Breakfast foods (Always provide protein with each meal or snack.)

- Eggs any style
- Fresh fruit and juices
- Gluten-Free cereal, hot or cold - add fresh fruit, raisins, nuts, or cinnamon for flavor, combined with milk of your choose or yogurt.
- Gluten-Free toast, bagels, pancakes or waffle, (usually found in the freezer or refrigerator sections). My favorite pancake mix company is Authentic Foods.
- Gluten-Free muffins, cornbread or similar baked goods. Combine with eggs, nut butter of your choose or yogurt.
- Gluten-Free yogurt with fresh fruit (coconut and goat yogurt are available)
- Gluten-Free Protein Shakes with fresh fruit, (There are protein powders that are dairy, casein and whey free)

Lunch

- Amy's Macs and Cheese: Amy's brand makes 2 types of GF Macs and Cheese with and without dairy.
- Burritos or tacos using brown rice tortilla or corn tortilla with choice of GF filling
- Fresh fruit and/or veggies with dips such as hummus or yogurt/dill dressing.
- Gluten-Free soup, chili, chowder (Several GF companies make canned soup & chili)
- Leftovers (make enough dinner for lunch leftovers)
- Gluten·Free Pizza (many restaurants now offer GF pizza, several GF companies made GF pizza crust – found in freezer section)
- Sandwich with Gluten-Free roll/ bread and Gluten-Free condiments. (Boar's Head meats are GF)
- Yogurt or Cottage cheese and fruit

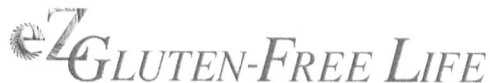

Some Frozen Meal available for kids
(New products become available frequently

Amy's Kid Meals
- Baked Ziti (GF & DF)
- Macs and Cheese
- Variety of Pizza

Ian's
- Chicken Nuggets
- Fish Sticks
- Variety Of Pizza
- Waffles

Always try to pair your meal or snack with a PROTEIN

Cheese	**Types of Cheeses**
	Almond
	Cow
	Goat
	Sheep
	Rice (Vegan rice cheese does not have Casein)
	Daiya Cheese: Gluten & Dairy Free
Deli Meats	Boar's Head, Hormel Deli, Applegate are GF
Edamame	
Meat	
Milk	**Types of Milk**
	Almond
	Cow
	Goat
	Rice
	Sheep
Nuts & Seeds	
Nuts Butters	
Soy nuts	
Yogurt	**Types of Yogurt**
	Almond Milk Yogurt
	Coconut Yogurt
	Cow Yogurt
	Goat Yogurt
	Sheep Yogurt
	Rice Yogurt

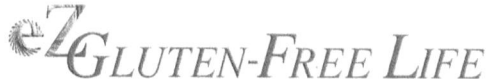

Healthy Snacks for Kids: Gluten Free

Fruit Ideas
All fruit can be cut in fun shapes
Canned fruit in its own syrup
ClifKidZ's fruit rope
Dole Fruit Cups
FruitaBü
Funky Monkey (Freeze-Dried Fruit)
Materno GoGo Squeeze (Applesauce)
Matt's Munchies Fruit Snacks
Peeled Snacks' dreid Fruit Picks
Rhythum Kale Chips
Seneca: Apple Chips
Sensible Foods dried fruit
Sensible Foods: Dried Fruit Snacks
Stretch Island Fruit co's (Fruit Strips)
Unsweetened apple sauce

Vegetable Ideas
Crunchies: Freeze Dried
           Veggies Snacks
Celery Sticks
Carrot sticks
Broccoli
Cucumbers
Dried Edamame
Dried Peas
snackLets: Kale Chips
Snapea Crisps
Soy nuts

Combined with Dips
GF Light Ranch Dressings

Guacamole
Hummus: Sabra is GF has single servings
Nut Butter

Healthy Snacks for Kids: Gluten Free

Alternative Snacks	Brands
Bagel Chips	El's kitchen
Baked Fries and/or Cheese Puffs	Snikiddy
Cereal: gluten-free	**There are many GF options**
(Send a bag of cereal to snack on)	Barbara's
	Chex
	Nature's Path EnviroKidz
Chips: gluten-free	Baked Lay's GF
(Beware of sodium and fat count)	
	Bearitos
	Food Should Taste Good Chips
	(single servings)
	Seneca Potato Chips
	Terra Chips
Crackers	Hol-Grain Brown Rice Crackers
	Mary's Gone Crackers
	Back to Nature Sesame Seed Rice Crackers
	Crunchmaster Crackers
Granola & Granola Bars	Udi's
	Enjoy Life
	Glutenfeeda and Bakery
	Bakery on Main
	Pamela's
Popcorn	Orville Redenbacher's *Natural* (dairy-free)
Pretzel's	Synder's of Hanover
	Glutino
	Dutch County Soft Pretzels (online)
Protein Bars:	**Kid Friendly Protein Bars**
(Beware of nut content, fiber, sugar and protein count)	Kind Bars
	Larabars
	Wholehealtheveryday.com
	(Homemade bars)
	Zing bars

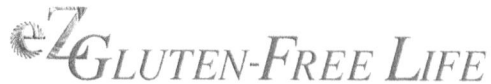

TREATS FOR THE FAMILY	BRAND NAMES
Baked Goods	1-2-3 Gluten Free
	Enjoy Life
	Jennies Gluten-Free Bakery
	Pamela's
	Three Senses Gourmet: GF Desserts
	(not dairy-free)
	Udi's Muffins (frozen)
Baked Mixes	1-2-3 Gluten Free
	Authentic Foods
	Better Batter
	Mina's Purely Divine
	Pamela's
Candy	See candy page
Cookies	Consenza
GF Cookie companies are not always dairy-free.	Cybeles: New company
Please read ingredients.	GinnyBakes
	Lucy's
	Mary's Go Crackers
	Mi-Del
	Pamela's
	Simply Shari's
	Trader Joes
	Udi's (boxed and frozen)
Chips	Baked Lays
	Corn Chips: Most corn chips are gluten-free, read ingredients to be sure
	Food Should Taste Good Chips
	Seneca Apple Chips
	Terra Chips

TREATS FOR THE FAMILY	BRAND NAMES

Chocolate
(Beware of malt barley in some chocolate)
Many chocolate products contain dairy.
If dairy is an issue then milk chocolate is out.
 	
Dark chocolate is often dairy-free.
Look for the words milk, non-fat milk,
milk powder, milk solids, casein, and butter.
Cocoa butter is dairy-free.
	Enjoy Life: Dairy and gluten-free bars
	    and chips (my favorite)
	Justin: GF & DF peanut butter cups
	    (so good)
	Rice Dream: Dairy and gluten-free bars
	and chips

Ice cream and Ice bars	Luna & Larry's Coconut Bliss: Excellent gluten-free and dairy-free ice cream Almond Dream: Very good dairy-free ice cream (Read labels -some products may share a machine with milk. Many of the flavors are gluten-free. (Lil'-Dreamers are NOT gluten-free) Rice Dream and Soy Dream: Products will have a gluten-free icon on them. Power of fruit: Frozen fruit bars that are 100% fruit and fruit juice
Marshmallows	Dandies: air puffed Marshmallows that are gluten-free and dairy-free and vegan.
Specialty Popcorn	479 Popcorn: Gluten-Free. Air popped treats in a bag. Bearitos Popcorn Paul Newman's Popcorn

FAST FOOD AT A GLANCE

For a detailed breakdown of gluten-free fast foods please refer to *Is Gluten Hiding in Unexpected Places*. (Coming soon)

Fast Foods with gluten-free options

(Possible Cross Contamination)

Chick-fil-A
In & Out Burger
Rubio's
Sonic Burgers

BEST fast foods with gluten-free options

(Possible Cross Contamination)

Arby's
Burger King
Chick-fil-A
DQ®
Jack in the box
McDonald's
Rubio's
Sonic Burger
Taco Bell
Wendy's

Fast Foods with FEW or NO gluten-free options

(Possible Cross Contamination)

Carl's Jr.
Del Taco
Domino's Pizza
El Pollo Loco
Fatburger
KFC
Panda Express
Pizza Hut
White Castle

Facts about Fast Food restaurants and a gluten-free menu:
1. The gluten-free food menu is for those that are gluten sensitive only and not Celiac's.
2. Cross contamination is extremely difficult to avoid.
3. Often fast food restaurants do not allow their employees to comment on allergen in the food.
4. Ingredients or production methods used by suppliers may change, or there may be product differences among regional suppliers.
5. Menus are continually changing. Please go to company website to review allergen menus.
6. The attached information has been updated in 2013, from the restaurants website or by personally contacting the company.

Below is an example of one fast food restaurant disclaimer and is a good representation of the disclaimers in the fast food industry:

"Gluten-Free" designations are based on information provided by our ingredient suppliers.

Warning:

Ingredients or production methods used by our suppliers may change, or there may be product differences among regional suppliers. Additionally, normal kitchen operations involve shared cooking and preparation areas, or we may need to substitute ingredients in menu items. We are therefore unable to guarantee that any menu item is free from gluten or any other allergen, and we assume no responsibility for guests with food allergies or sensitivities.

*eZ*GLUTEN-FREE LIFE

Fast Food at a Glance: The French Fries	GF	DF	GLUTEN
Arby's			
Curly Fries			GLUTEN
Homestyle Fries			GLUTEN
Burger King	GF	DF	
Regular Fries	GF	DF	
Sweet Potato Fries	GF	DF	
Carl's Jr.			
Chili Cheese Fries			GLUTEN
Criss Cross Fries			GLUTEN
Regular Fries	GF	DF	
Chick-fil-A			
Waffle Potato	GF	DF	
Del Taco			GLUTEN
Chili Cheese Fries			GLUTEN
Deluxe Chili Cheese Fries			GLUTEN
Regular Fries	GF	DF	
DQ®			GLUTEN
French Fries	GF	DF	
Chili Fries	GF		
Fatburger			
Fat Fries	GF	DF	
Chile Fries	GF		
In & Out Burger	GF	DF	
Jack in the box		DF	GLUTEN
McDonald's			GLUTEN
KFC			
Potato Wedges		DF	GLUTEN
Pizza Hut			
Taters	GF	DF	
Sonic Burger	GF	DF	
Wendy's			GLUTEN
White Castle	GF	DF	

For a complete list of Fast Foods Gluten-Free menus please refer to *Is Gluten Hiding in Unexpected Places*. (Coming soon)

Menus and ingredients in restaurants change often, please ask for confirmation that food is gluten-free whenever you eat out.

VERIFIED 2013

DAIRY	DEDICATED FRYER
	NO
	NO
DAIRY	NO
	NO
	NO
	NO
	NO
DAIRY	NO
	NO
	NO
	NO
	NO
	NO
DAIRY	NO
DAIRY	NO
	NO
	NO
	NO
DAIRY	NO
	NO
	NO
DAIRY	NO
	YES
	NO
DAIRY	NO
	NO
	NO
	NO
	NO
DAIRY	NO
	NO

Please see "Page 5" for disclaimer.

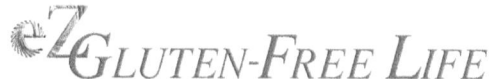

CANDY AT A GLANCE

Below is a list of candy brands and/or companies. The list is divided by 100% gluten-free, some items are gluten-free, possible cross contaminations, no gluten-free options, or the company requests the consumer reads ingredient labels. For specific details please request my Candy Handbook.

Brands and/or Companies that are 100% gluten-free
Annies
Ce De Candy (Smarties)
Crispy Cats
Enjoy Life
Ferrara Pan (Gummy bears etc)
Jelly Bellys
Pearson's (Salted Nut Rolls, Mint Patties, Nut Goodies and Bun Bars)
Surf Sweets (Gummy Worms Etc)
Toostie (All except Andes Cookies)
Yummy Earth

Brands that have some gluten-free options
Annabelle
Cadbury Adams
HERSHEY'S
Impact Confection's (Warheads)
Just Born (MIKE AND IKE®,HOT TAMALE®, PEEPS®, GOLDENBERG'S PEANUT CHEWS®, TEENEE NEANEE® AND JUST BORN® BRANDS HAVE SOME GF ITEMS)
NECCO
NESTLES® (Some items)
NESTLES WONKA® (Some items)
See's Candy (Candy Canes, Climber Canes, Puppet Candy Sticks, Thanksgiving Chocolate Cream)
Spangler Candy

Brands that are gluten-free but may be exposed to cross contamination
Airhead
Russell Stover

Brands that are not gluten-free
Godiva

A brand that does not have a gluten-free list and request the consumer read ingredient labels
Mars

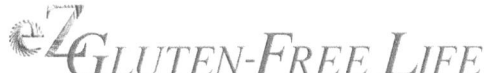
Acknowledgements

When you see the name of an author on the book it is only telling part of the story. Behind every author is a host of friends, family, and professionals who have given of themselves so that the author could write this book. It takes a community which inspires, encourages, guides, educates and loves the author through the process.

Dr. Cynthia Costa, thank you for my renewed health and your guidance. I remember the day Dr. Costa diagnosed me with Hashimoto's. She came into the office and leaned against the door frame. "You may never be able to eat certain foods ever again", she quietly stated as if this were a life sentence. I thought, "If that is all I have to do then bring it on." And bring it on she did. The diagnosis and eliminating gluten, dairy, soy and other foods not only improved my quality of life dramatically, it also ignited a passion in me for learning everything I could about gluten, living gluten-free, and helping others in the process. Thank you for suggesting that I become a gluten-free consultant and asking me whether or not there is gluten in numerous products. I am so grateful that Dr. Costa is my doctor, business associate, and friend.

Wendy Meg Siegel's existence defines my word for gratitude. She is my dearest and longest friend. Thank you for always being there for me. Thank you for believing in me, even when I did not believe in myself. Thank you for all your love and continued support. Thank you for your time; I know how precious it is.

My brother, Michael, is a true miracle in this journey I have been on. He is the graphic artist who designed my logo, titles of my companies, and created the blueprint for my handbooks. I cannot begin to adequately describe the endless hours he has spent helping me develop this business. He has given of his time, his talent, and his love to take my visions and make them a reality. I will be forever grateful.

My dear husband, Richard, is my rock. He loves me unconditionally, he believes in me completely, and he is always there for me.

My daughter Alexandria's birth showed me dreams do come true. She continues to inspire me every day.

I love you all!

NOTES:

NOTES:

NOTES:

NOTES: